DOGGY STYLE
SEX
FOR ONE WEEK

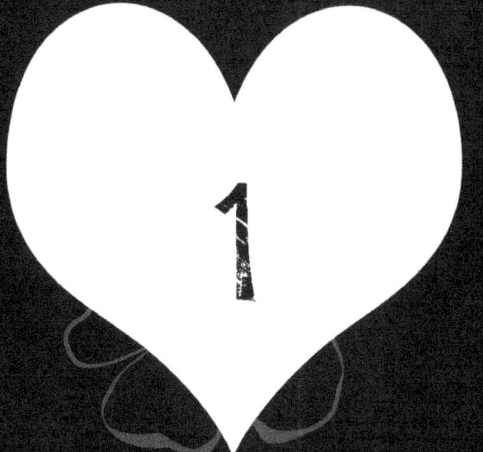

1

BACKSIDE OF COUPON

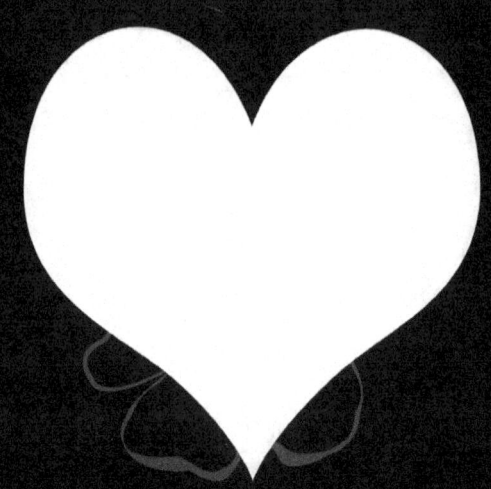

VALENTINE SEX COUPONS

Cupid Love

ISBN: 10: 1542581982
ISBN-13: 978-1542581981

Do You Want More Sex Coupons in Your Email and new and fun sex ideas go to SexVouchers.Com And sign up for our email list.

TEAR OUT
COUPONS TO REDEEM

69
SIDEWAYS 69
REVERSE 69

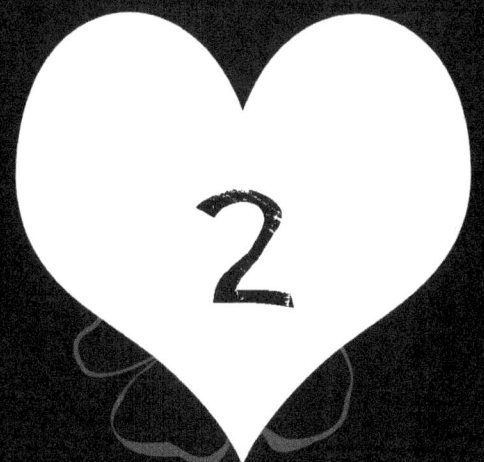
2

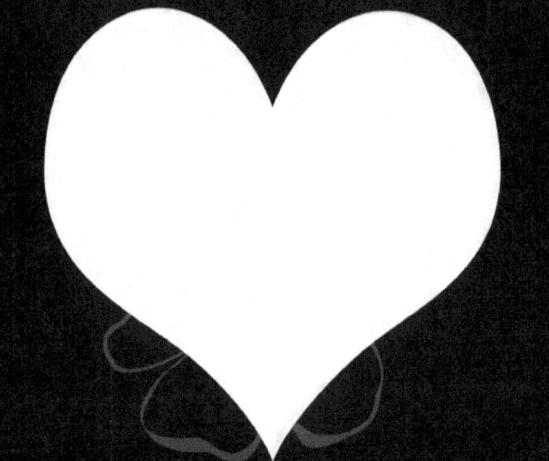

BACKSIDE OF COUPON

My Favorite Sex Position For 3 Days

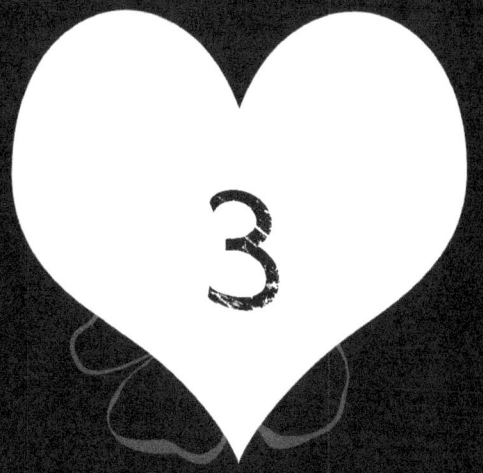

3

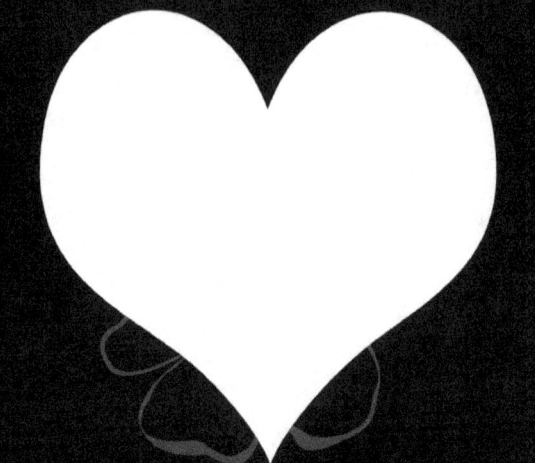

BACKSIDE OF
COUPON

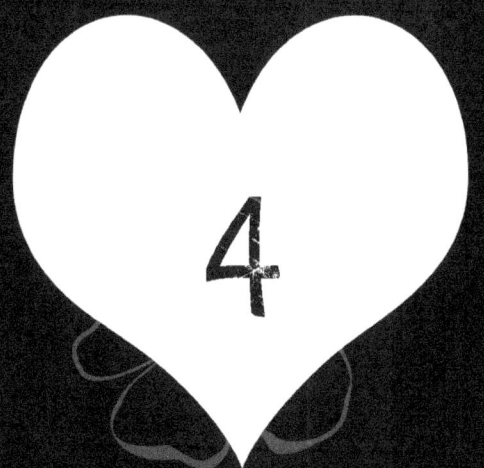

FUCK ME HARD AND QUICK

4

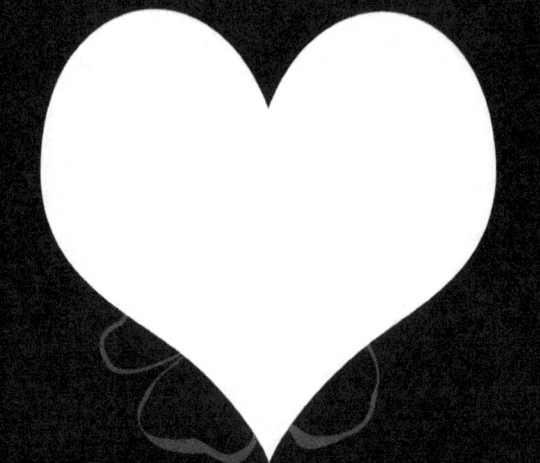

BACKSIDE OF COUPON

Reverse Cow Girl For One Day Every 2 Hours

5

BACKSIDE OF COUPON

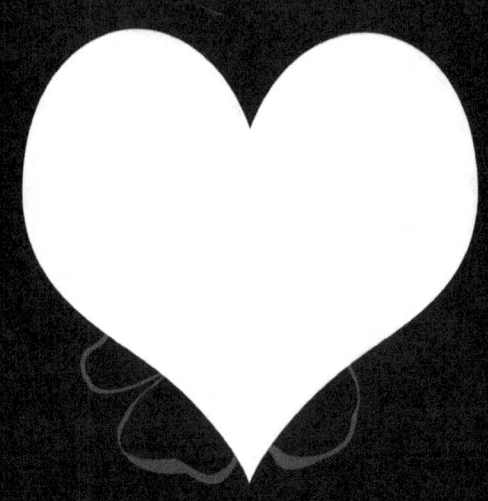

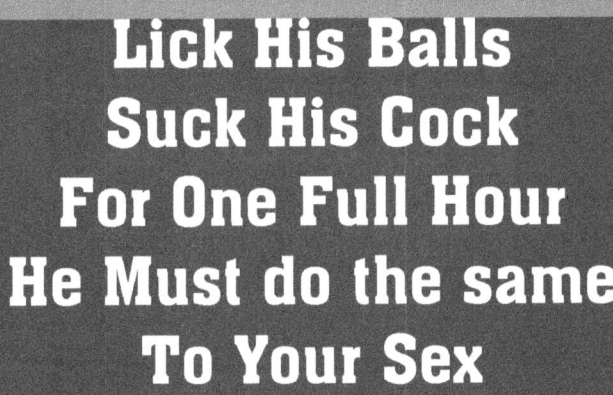

Lick His Balls
Suck His Cock
For One Full Hour
He Must do the same
To Your Sex

6

BACKSIDE OF COUPON

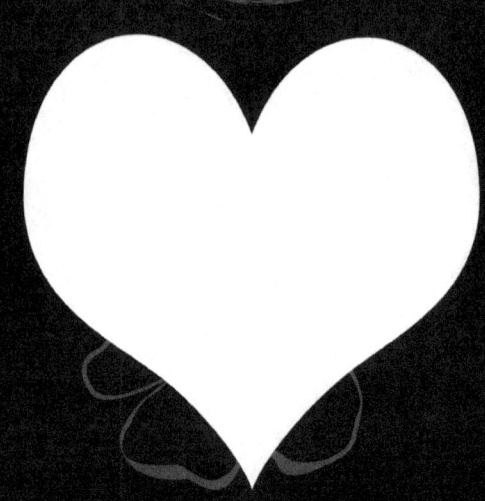

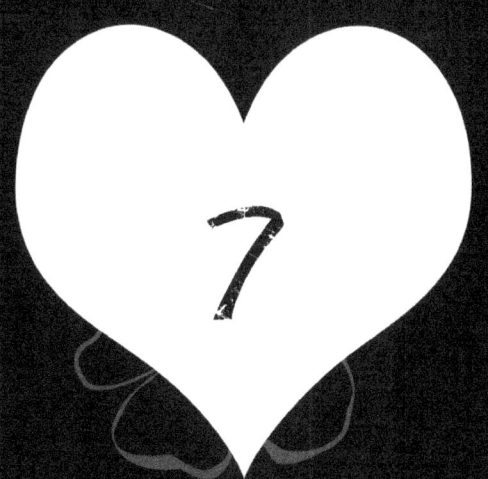

Use an Anal Sex Toy On Her While You Have Doggy Style Sex Make sure you use lube

7

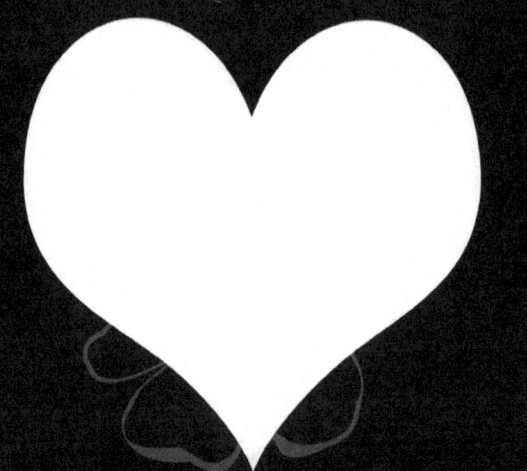

BACKSIDE OF COUPON

Tonight you get to tie each other up and have your way with your lover. Switch after one hour

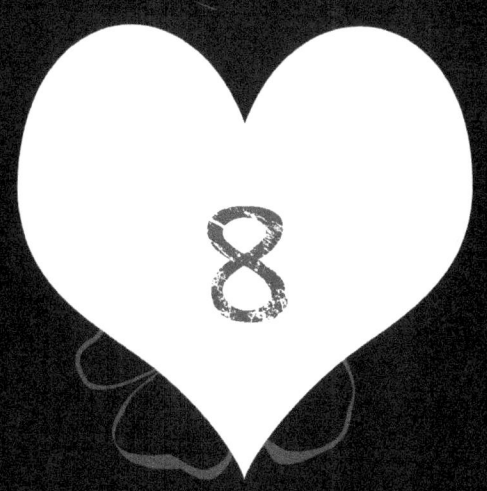

BACKSIDE OF COUPON

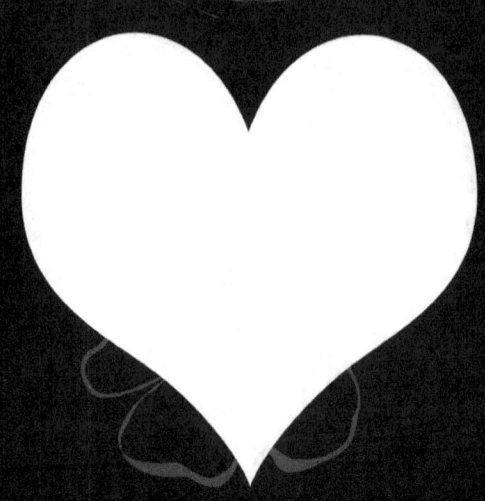

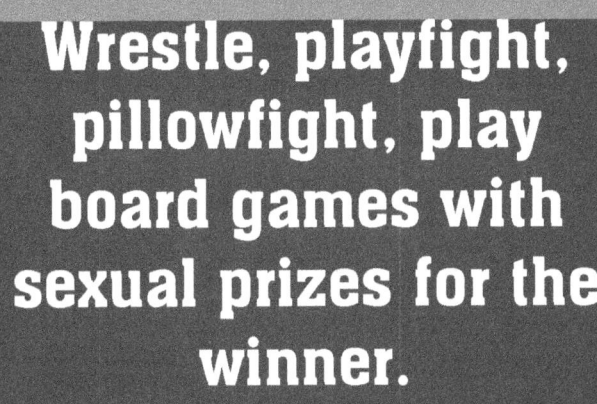

Wrestle, playfight, pillowfight, play board games with sexual prizes for the winner.

9

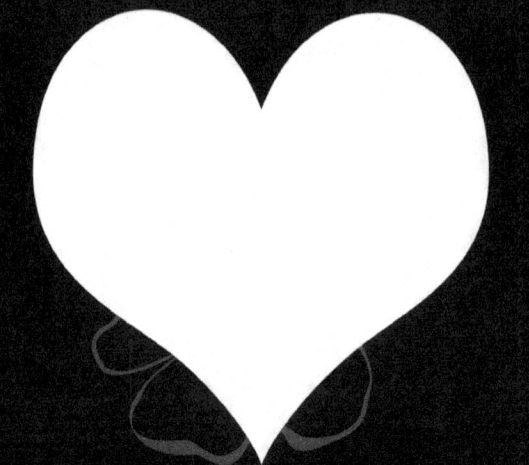

BACKSIDE OF COUPON

Sex In Every room of the house. A different room, with a different position.

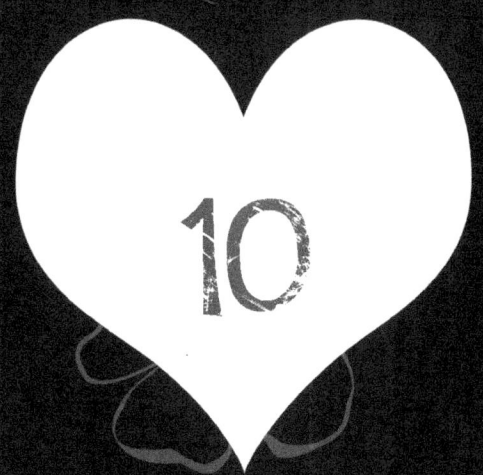

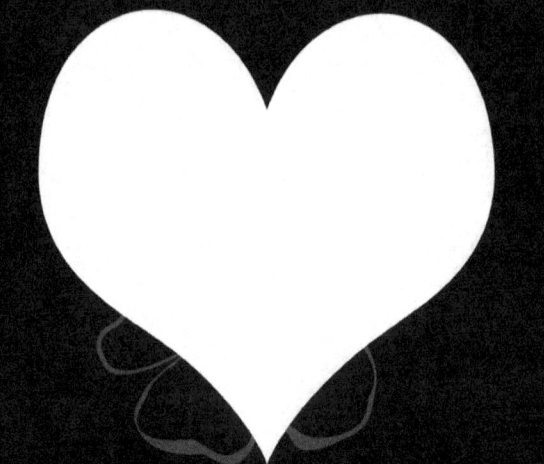

BACKSIDE OF COUPON

A 45 Minute Massage for each person with hand or mouth happy ending for each person.

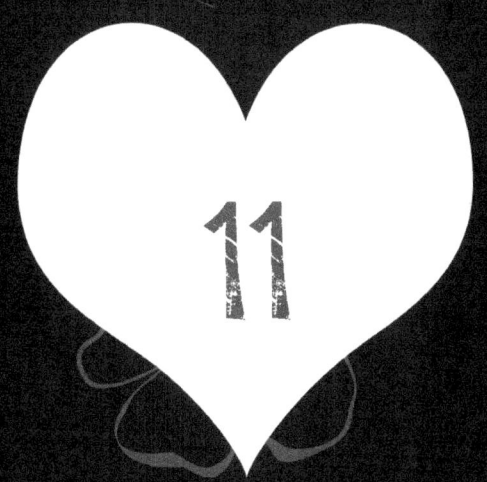

11

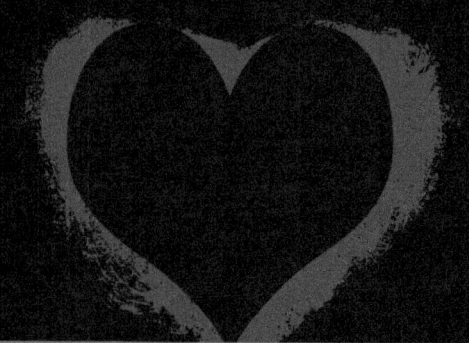

BACKSIDE OF COUPON

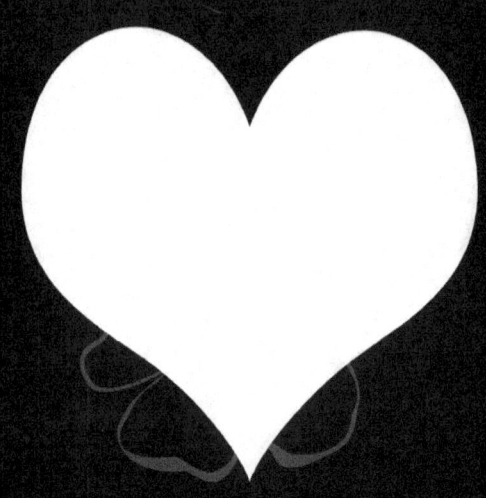

Roleplay: He is a patient and she is the sexy nurse that must take away his aches and pains.

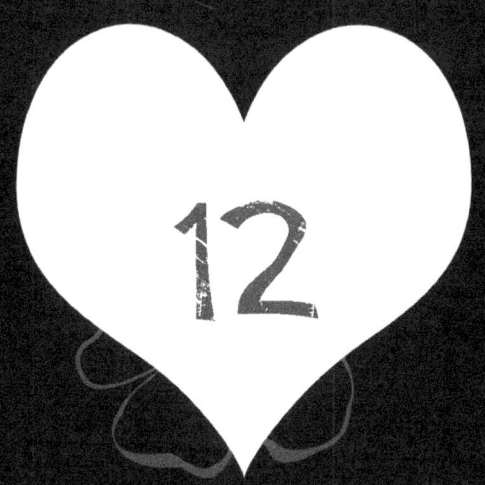

12

BACKSIDE OF COUPON

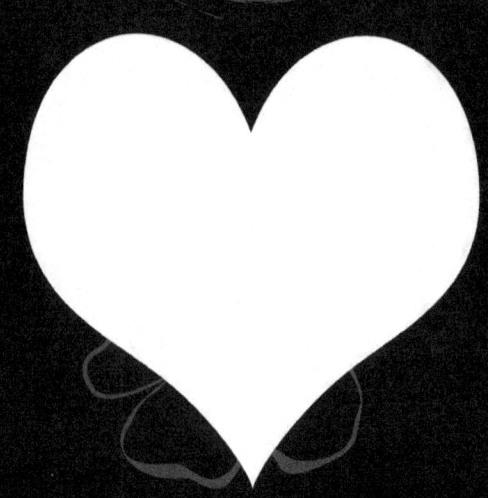